Overcoming Dyslexia

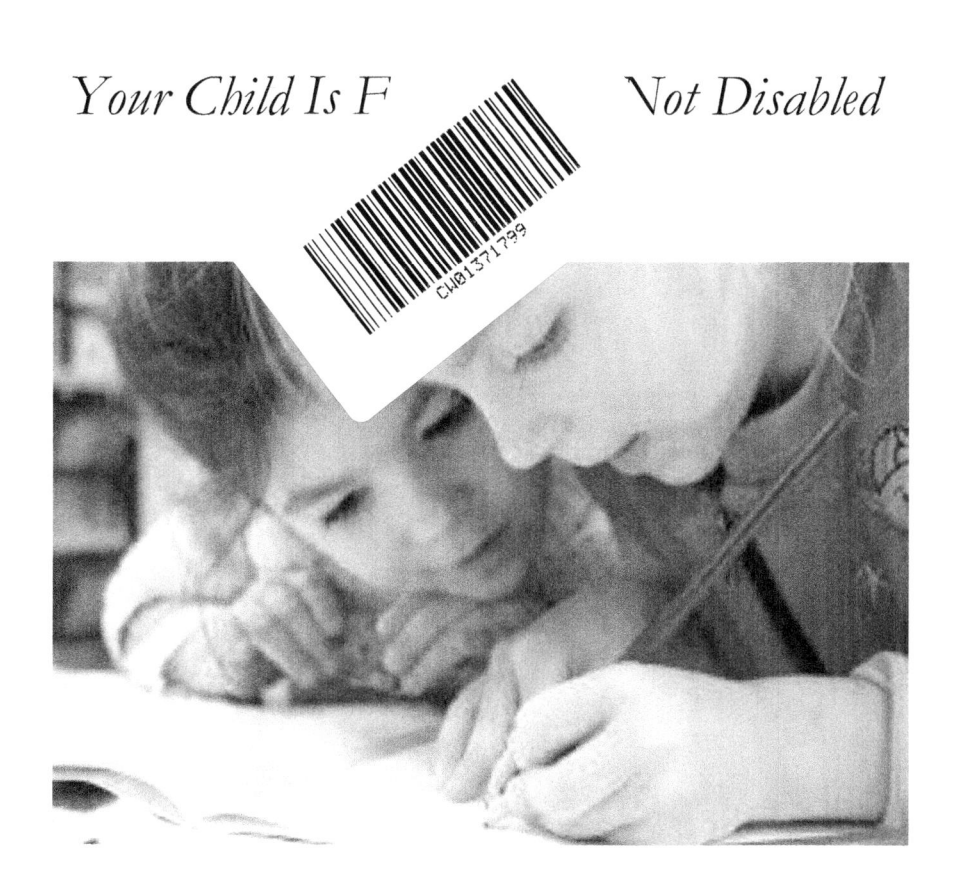

Your Child Is F̶ ̶N̶ot Disabled

Jimmy D. Forest

Bluesource And Friends

This book is brought to you by Bluesource And Friends, a happy book publishing company.

Our motto is **"Happiness Within Pages"**

We promise to deliver amazing value to readers with our books. We also appreciate honest book reviews from our readers.

Connect with us on our Facebook page www.facebook.com/bluesourceandfriends and stay tuned to our latest book promotions and free giveaways.

Don't forget to claim your FREE books!

Brain Teasers:

https://tinyurl.com/karenbrainteasers

Harry Potter Trivia:

https://tinyurl.com/wizardworldtrivia

Sherlock Puzzle Book (Volume 2)

https://tinyurl.com/Sherlockpuzzlebook2

Also check out our best seller book
"67 Lateral Thinking Puzzles"

https://tinyurl.com/thinkingandriddles

Table of Contents

Table of Contents

Introduction

Chapter 1: Overview Of Learning Disabilities

   Facts about Learning Disabilities

Chapter 2: Does Your Child Have Dyslexia and What Are the Symptoms?

Chapter 3: Comparing Dyslexia and ADHD

   Summary of Differences between ADHD and Dyslexia

   Types of Dyslexia

   Possible Causes of Dyslexia

Chapter 4: Diagnosing Dyslexia

   Symptoms in Preschoolers

   Symptoms in Grade Schoolers

   Symptoms in Older Children

Chapter 5: Inability To Read Doesn't Mean Your Kid Is Dumb

Chapter 6: Managing Parents' Emotions and Expectations

Chapter 7: Your Child Just Needs to Learn Differently

Chapter 8: Test a Fish in Swimming but Not Climbing a Tree

Chapter 9: Self-Awareness and Acceptance for Kids with Dyslexia

Chapter 10: Helping Your Child Breakthrough In Reading

Simplified Steps

Gradually Introduce Harder Books

Choosing the Books to Read

Handwriting

Chapter 11: Helping Your Child Breakthrough In Math

Techniques to Help a Dyslexic Child with Math

Using the Senses

Using Auditory Skills

Chapter 12: Seeking Therapy

Chapter 13: Joining a Support Group (Actually Helps)

Finding the Right Group

Making a Financial Plan

Chapter 14: Summary: Ways a Parent can help a Dyslexic Child at Home

Helping the Dyslexic Child with Organization

Helping a Dyslexic Child with Spelling

Helping a Dyslexic Child with Writing

Helping a Child with Reading

Helping Your Child with Memory

Conclusion

Introduction

Congratulations on getting *Overcoming dyslexia* and thank you for doing so. Dyslexia is a learning disability that is more common than most people think. It is a multifaceted and complex diagnosis that was seen as untreatable for many decades. In this book, we will take you through the basics of dyslexia in children, how to identify it, and the ways that a parent can help the child. This book take you through the stages from when you as a parent or guardian start to think that the child has a problem, identify the exact problem, finding the most appropriate treatment, and helping the child to transition from 'learning to read' to 'reading to learn,' and later, into the real world.

The most important thing is to know that there are interventions and therapies that can help the child to acquire ether literacy skills that seem hard. With the right techniques and support, the child can learn how to spell, read, and write. A dyslexic child is as intelligent and curious as any other child; therefore he/she stands as good a chance as any other to pursue their dreams and goals. This book aims to help parents improve the situation of their kids and getting them back on track.

To that end, Chapter 1 will cover an overview of learning disabilities, Chapter 2, the symptoms of dyslexia, Chapter 3, a comparison of dyslexia and ADHD, Chapter 4, how to dragonize dyslexia, Chapter

5, dyslexia does not mean dumbness, Chapter 6, managing emotions and Chapter 7, a dyslexic child has to learn differently. Chapter 8 will explain how to identify the strengths of a child, Chapter 9, self-awareness and acceptance, Chapter 10 and 11 will focus on how to help a kid breakthrough in reading and math, Chapter 12 will talk about seeking therapy, Chapter 13 will address joining a support group, and Chapter 14 will summarize the ways to help a dyslexic child.

Chapter 1: Overview Of Learning Disabilities

The term "Learning Disability" refers to neurologically based processing challenges. These challenges normally interfere with the basic skills of learning how to read, write, spell and do math related processes. Some of them also interrupt the higher level skills such as time management, organization, memory, abstract reasoning, et cetera. It is important to note that learning disabilities can affect a person beyond the learning spectrum and impact the relationship with other people.

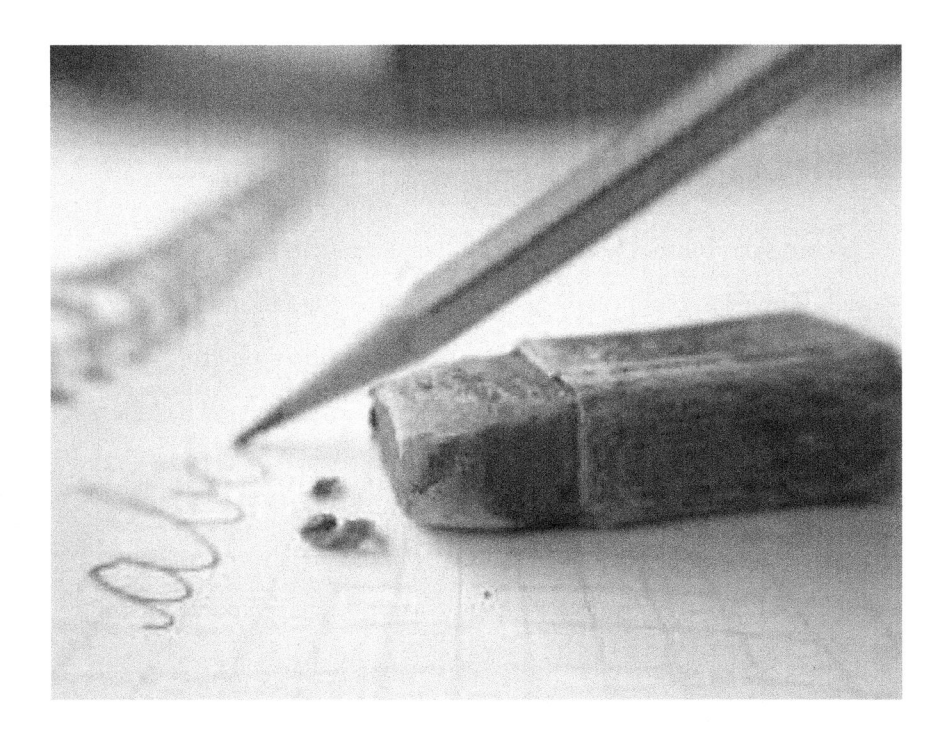

Challenges with reading, spelling, writing or math can be recognized at an early age, but some people go undiagnosed until their adult life. Learning disabilities do not refer to the same thing as learning problems. Normally, learning problems result from hearing, visual, or motor handicap.

Generally speaking, people who have learning disabilities have an average or above average level of intelligence. In most cases, there appears to be a ridge between the potential of the affected individual and the actual achievement. Consequently, learning disabilities are also termed as hidden disabilities; the person seems perfectly normal, with high levels of intelligence and brightness, but he/she is unable to demonstrate the level of skills expected from someone of corresponding age.

A learning disability is a lifelong challenge that cannot be fixed or cured. However, technology and research have led to interventions that can help a child to achieve as much as a normal person. With the right support and intervention, any person can achieve all he/she dreams of regardless of the challenge.

Facts about Learning Disabilities

Research shows that there is a genetic component linked to learning disabilities.

Learning disabilities are life long and cannot be outgrown. However, the affected person can learn to compensate for the difficulties; therefore, early diagnosis is recommended.

Learning disabilities cannot be diagnosed through medical tests like blood tests, but it can be diagnosed by a trained professional after careful testing and evaluation of the child.

There is a wrong assumption that has been associated with learning disabilities. Many people assume that they occur due to cognitive delays. This is not true. It has been found that many people know that dyslexia affects learning, but not many people can define the condition clearly. As such, many people think that ADHD and dyslexia are one condition with similar treatments.

Chapter 2: Does Your Child Have Dyslexia And What Are the Symptoms?

Dyslexia

The majority of people think that dyslexia is a rare problem, but they are wrong. Reading ability does not come easily and naturally to everyone. In fact, you will be surprised to find that many girls and boys, including some of the very bright and talented ones, have a challenging time learning how to read. For reading beginners, this condition involves the inability to manipulate or notice the sounds in a spoken word. Consequently, this deficiency affects the accuracy of reading, the reading rate, and also spelling. A child is able to link letters to sounds after he develops an awareness of the sounds of the spoken words. From this development, the child sounds out new words. The dyslexic children face a challenge in making this development; therefore, they need extra help to break the reading code. Normally, children with dyslexia have terrible handwriting because their hands have trouble making out letters.

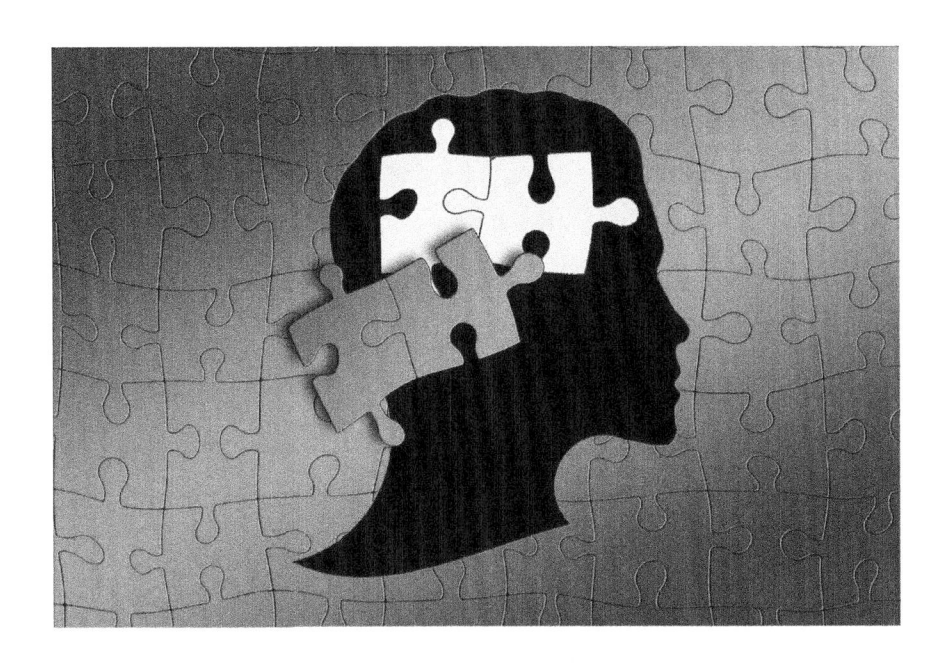

Dyslexia refers to a condition where people have a harder time reading and writing than other people. The term dyslexia comes from two Greek words: 'dys' which means ill, and 'lexia' referring to word. Although the statistics are not clear about the number of children suffering from dyslexia, it is the most common issue affecting learning. Some people believe that this condition is a visual issue, whereby the kid reads or writes the letters backward, but it is not. Dyslexia issue is not a vision challenge, nor is it seeing lettered in the wrong direction. It is also important to note that dyslexia is not an intelligence problem even though it impacts learning. Children with such issues are as intelligent as their peers, and many people have gotten successful careers even after struggling with reading and writing.

The worst myth that makes most people ignore the dyslexic children is the assumption that the young ones will outgrow the problem. They assume that it is just a hurdle with reading as a skill. Dyslexia is not outgrown. As such, the child has to get help as soon as possible.

Signs and Symptoms

Dyslexia affects people in varying degrees and as such, the symptoms vary for different children. The most common sign that might signal a child is struggling with reading and writing is find a challenge learning and enjoying the common nursery rhymes such as Jack & Jill. This refers to children aged three and above. They have a hard time recognizing that the common link in the Cat in the Hat rhyme is 'at.' As time goes by, the child may have a challenge recognizing the sounds or names of letters in the alphabet. In this case, we are not talking about knowing the ABC song; rather it's about identifying and knowing the name of a letter and then the sound it makes such as 'em' for M. The child may even be unable to write or read their own name.

Statistics show that one on every five children is dyslexic. Sadly, most of them are mistaken for being stupid or lazy because most people do not understand dyslexia. When a child has a hard time reading, life becomes very hard, especially in the current world; the ability and inability to read affects all aspects of life directly or indirectly, including self-esteem. In most cases, the condition of dyslexia goes undiagnosed in children until they are into elementary school, and at this juncture, it is harder to address. However, scientists have found that reading challenges can be spotted in early childhood. When diagnosed early enough, and with the right support, there are high chances that the struggling leaders will learn how to be good readers.

A recent study conducted by scientists at Yale University School of Medicine found that when young children are taught solid skills on connecting sounds with letters (decoding) early on, and get intensive and prompt help in learning spelling, comprehension and vocabulary skills, they can master the required reading skills. In fact, through comparing different brain scans, the research found that the struggling readers who received intense help had a stimulated reading system.

Co-Occurrences
One of the main reasons why a child should undergo a full evaluation that assesses all areas of learning when being tested for dyslexia, involves ruling out all other conditions that might have almost the same symptoms. There are a number of issues that occur alongside dyslexia, and many kids tend to have more than one attention and learning issue. Some of the issues that may be mistaken or co-occur with dyslexia include:

ADHD (Attention Deficiency Hyperactivity Disorder): Can make it tough for children to stay focused in most activities including reading. An estimated 40% of children with ADHD also have dyslexia. However, the kids with dyslexia will most likely act out or fidget in class because of the frustration of reading unlike those with ADHD.

Executive Functioning Issues: These issues affect different areas and skills of learning. Some of the executive functioning includes flexible thinking, organization, and working memory.

Slow Processing Speed: Another issue that might be mistaken for Dyslexia is slow processing speed, which impacts the reading ability. Children suffering from this issue have a harder time taking in, processing, and responding to information. As such, they have a challenge mastering basic reading skills and grasping the meaning of the things they have read.

Auditory Processing Disorder (APD): This issue involves difficulties in sorting through the sounds that one hears. Consequently, APD makes it hard for an individual to recognize the difference between the sounds of letters and sounding new words.

Visual Processing Issues: This involves the challenges of making out the things that the eyes see. The kids suffering from visual processing issues may complain that the letters are blurry or are 'hopping around on the page.' In an attempt to compensate for the visual challenges, the affected children compensate by closing one eye or squinting. They also tend to write letters in reverse and have a hard time staying within the lines. Dyslexic children also have these symptoms and similar complaints.

Dyscalculia: This condition makes it hard for one to do math. A majority of the kids that have a challenge reading and doing math may have dyscalculia co-occurring with Dyslexia. It is therefore very important to diagnose the condition accurately.

Dysgraphia: This affects the ability of the child to spell, and form numbers and letters. The kids suffering from this condition also have a hard time organizing thoughts on paper. This condition often co-occurs with dyslexia.

Chapter 3: Comparing Dyslexia and ADHD

It can be difficult to tell whether dyslexia or Attention Deficiency Hyperactivity Disorder is causing a child to be distracted, inattentive, or have difficulties reading, following instructions, and writing. In some cases, the two conditions co-occur. Statistics show that one out of every four children with Attention Deficiency Hyperactivity Disorder also has dyslexia. Again, between 15% and 40% of kids with dyslexia also have ADHD. Both conditions require the child and his/her family to work together in order to manage the conditions.

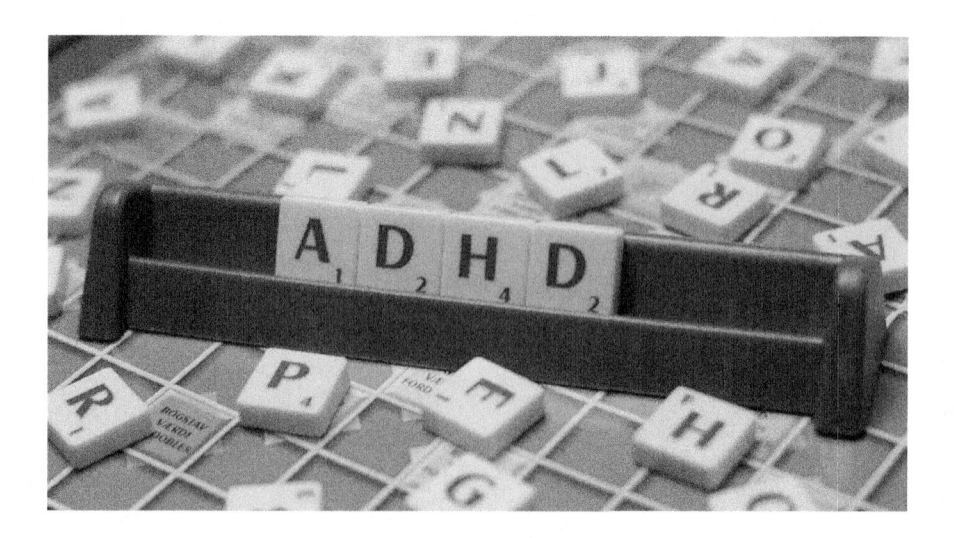

Differentiating between Dyslexia and ADHD may seem like a tough task, especially for the people that have no experience with the condition. When reading, does the child skip words because he/she cannot pronounce, them or is it that he/she is reading too fast and missing some words? In the world, ADHD is making more headlines than dyslexia; therefore a parent will be tempted to associate slowness in reading with ADHD. It is, however, very important for one to assess the writing and reading difficulties from all angles. ADHD is more inclined toward behavioral challenges, while Dyslexia is highly restricted to reading and writing. Despite the differences, there are some observable links between the two conditions. Scientists have found that both disorders involve similar areas of the brain. The two conditions appear to cause problems in the memory, executive functioning, and processing of symbols quickly. The affected children will appear distracted, lack fluency, and have problems when writing. These conditions also show a similarity in that they affected children normally have higher levels of creativity and intelligence, yet they are frustrated when it comes to academics.

The symptoms of dyslexia are exacerbated by ADHD and vice versa. The biggest challenge is that ADHD can be spotted from day one in school, while dyslexia might be missed until the child gets to grades that require the child to focus on 'reading to learn' rather than 'learning to read' (Normally fourth/fifth grade).

Summary of Differences between ADHD and Dyslexia

With dyslexia, the child will display attention and concentration problems primarily when reading and writing, but hardly in other situations. On the other hand, ADHD will be evident if the child has attention and concentration problems in any unstimulating task or environment.

Normally, the children with dyslexia will be better at auditory processing than the one with Attention Deficiency Hyperactivity Disorder. It is important to check and assess a child as soon as a parent or teacher sees the signs of any condition. so that they can start treatment in time. Delayed treatment for any of the conditions makes it worse and harder for the child to develop in the appropriate way.

The two conditions normally affect the self-esteem of the child if he/she is not guided well. It becomes a challenge for the child to feel good about him/herself when there are notable differences between him/her and peers, especially on tasks that are easy. There are some things that one may do to help the child build self-esteem and confidence, including:

Appreciating effort more than results: For the children with these conditions, it is advisable to appreciate efforts rather than grades or results. Children with dyslexia or Attention Deficiency Hyperactivity

Disorder have to work harder than the other kids, yet it might not reflect in the results or grades. It makes a lot of difference for the child if he/she realizes that their efforts are appreciated more than the results.

Identify: It is better if the child knows his/her condition by name. Although the parent may be uncomfortable giving the condition a name, it is advisable to let a child know what he/she is suffering from. Consequently, the child will stop looking for explanations as to why they are different from their peers and actually drop self-labels such as 'I am dumb.'

Activities: When a child shows interest in a positive activity, encourage it. Let the child be good at something, be it sports, martial arts, crafts, or anything that will build their confidence. Achievements in the areas of interest will create a ripple effect on the other sectors of life.

Types of Dyslexia

There are different types of dyslexia and a child may suffer from one or more. One child may be diagnosed with a dyslexia type where he/she has problems with sounds, while another person may have challenges with word and letter arrangement. To ensure that the child is diagnosed correctly, the specialists have classified dyslexia into different categories: surface dyslexia, phonological dyslexia, rapid naming deficit, and double deficit dyslexia.

Surface dyslexia is the condition where an individual has a problem understanding a word once he/she sees it. It is also referred to as visual dyslexia.

Phonological dyslexia refers to challenges where the individual has a problem putting sounds to letters when making up a word.

Rapid Naming dyslexia refers to the inability to name letters and numbers quickly.

Double deficit dyslexia refers to the combination of the rapid naming deficit and phonological dyslexia.

Possible Causes of Dyslexia

Researches have not yet pinpointed the exact cause of dyslexia, but there is some knowledge that brain and gene differences have a role to play. Some of the possible causes of dyslexia include:

Brain Anatomy and Activity: Studies conducted through brain imaging have revealed differences between the brains of people with and without dyslexia. The differences are mostly observed in the areas of the brain that deal with key reading abilities. The key skills in reading include knowing how words and sounds are represented, and recognizing the look of written words. Studies show that the brain can change. With the right tutoring, the brain activities of a dyslexic child can change.

Genes and Heredity: It has been observed that dyslexia sometimes runs in the families. Studies have found that about 40% of the siblings of children with dyslexia have the same reading challenges. Researches have also revealed that almost 49% of parents whose kids have dyslexia have it too. Scientists have also identified a number of genes that directly link to reading and processing issues.

Chapter 4: Diagnosing Dyslexia

One of the main challenges with dyslexia is that it can be hard to identify or spot until the child starts preschool. Even in school, the teachers and parents may make assumptions about the child and think that the difficulties will go away. A parent or teacher may at first notice struggles with reading, spelling, and following instructions that are easy for other kids of a similar age. The symptoms change as the child grows older; therefore, it is important that the parent and teacher understand what dyslexia looks like for different kids. Although children are different, there are some common symptoms that indicate the need for extra help getting along with the read, write, spell techniques.

Symptoms in Preschoolers

Children with dyslexia have challenges with phonetics, and as such, they lag behind their peers in term so f language skills. They will generally take longer to read, speak, and write than their friends and will sometimes get words and letters mixed up.

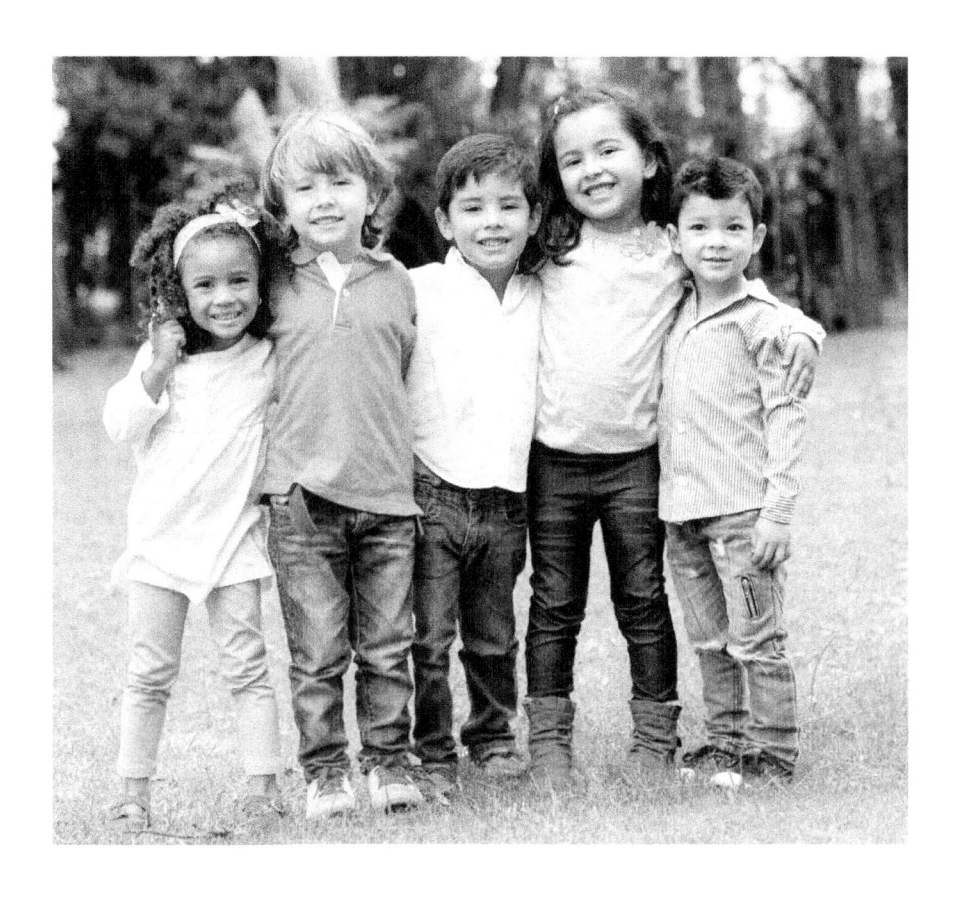

Preschoolers who have dyslexia will find it hard to remember the letters and numbers, they will mispronounce words that have similarities, for instance, pear and bear, or busgetti for spaghetti. They will do a lot of baby talk while they should be outgrowing it, and they may also have a hard time recognizing the rhyming patterns such as Humpty Dumpty on the wall, Humpty Dumpty took a fall.

Symptoms in Grade Schoolers

Among the grade schoolers, the symptoms of dyslexia will be more obvious, because the kids with the condition will have a harder time reading and writing than their classmates.

Grade schoolers with dyslexia will read at a slower pace than their peers; have a hard time telling the difference between certain words and letters; fail to connect the sounds and the letters like 'em' for 'm' and 'buh' for 'b'; write numbers or letters backward like 'b' instead of 'd' and '6' instead of '9'; write slowly; have a harder time understanding what they read; misspell even the simple words like 'and,' 'cat,' and 'dog'; say that the words on the page are dancing around; and struggle to follow instructions.

Symptoms in Older Children

Due to fear and embarrassment, young children may find ways to hide their literacy challenge when younger, but as they get older, it becomes hard to cover the weaknesses. The demands on the child increase and the child will find it more challenging to communicate with the peers. They might withdraw socially.

Middle and high school kids with dyslexia will have a challenge writing clearly (handwriting, grammar, punctuation, and spelling); take a longer time to complete tasks or homework; speak slowly; use wrong words like lotion for ocean, furnish for finish, etc.; avoid reading aloud; and constantly forget words and therefore keep saying 'um' or 'uh.'

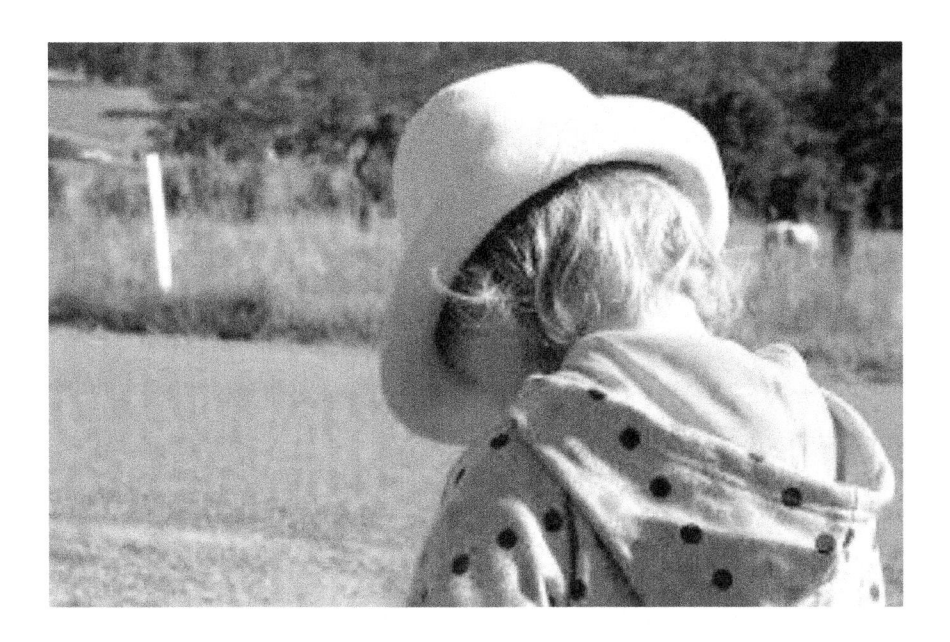

If a child shows these symptoms, it is important that the parent checks with the teachers in order to find out the progress in school. Many people might suspect that their child has dyslexia, but without the right diagnosis, one might not be able to tell for sure. The only way to get a sure answer is to take the child through a full evaluation, either privately or at school. Generally, school evaluations are free and having a sure diagnosis, also referred to as identification, allows a child to get the services and support he/she needs in life. These services may include specialized instructions and guidance in reading.

However, before one takes a child through the diagnosis process, it is important that they rule out any other medical issues, such as hearing and vision problems that might play a role in the child's condition.

There are a number of professionals who can assess kids for dyslexia, and they include school psychologists, pediatric neuropsychologists, and clinical psychologists. The evaluator will give the child a series of tests to check for dyslexia. In addition, the evaluator will assess other areas to identify where the weakness lies. A psychologist will look for other challenges that might be hindering the learning skills, for instance, mental issues and ADHD. This assessment will also include identifying if the child has co-occurring conditions. Besides that, the evaluator may ask for family history in order to identify the genesis of the condition.

Chapter 5: Inability To Read Doesn't Mean Your Kid Is Dumb

The inability or difficulty in reading resulting from dyslexia does not indicate that the child is dumb. In fact, dyslexic children are as smart as their fellow peers, and in some cases, they are above average. The best route to understanding dyslexia is to think of the condition as a state where the brain works differently, and therefore, the need for alternative tools to help the affected person to take in and hold the information that is taken by others quite simply.

There is nothing thick or deficient in kids with dyslexia. If anything, their brains work in a unique, special, and magical way. Dyslexia is actually a neurobiological glitch. Meaning, it is a functional variation found in the brain that makes it harder for the affected children to read. Scientists explain that the people with dyslexia tend to rely on their right brain more than the left. The right side is liable for creativity, holistic thoughts, music, art, and intuition while the left side hosts the language, logic, science, math, and analytical thought. For the dyslexic children, reading a word takes a longer trip through the brain. It is more challenging when such a child tries to read a sentence or a paragraph. This condition has been rooted in the phonological processing; the understanding of oral language, the otherwise simple process of identifying and blending sounds, rhyming, segmenting words, et cetera.

Kids with dyslexia may be tempted to feel that they are not as intelligent as their peers, because they have a difficult time keeping up. These problems can get worse as the children go through elementary school. In fact, the kids will look for ways to avoid reading because of stress and hardship. Consequently, they fall behind their peers in class because they miss valuable learning sessions. It is important that the parent and guardian focus on supporting the efforts of the child by assisting and encouraging them to read and write. Besides, the child should be given the opportunities to build confidence and succeed in other areas, for instance arts, sports, hobbies, and drama.

Chapter 6: Managing Parents' Emotions and Expectations

Every parent has high expectations for their child. There is hope so high that it seems more like an assumption, whereby the parent believes that the child will have a normal life, normal studying processes, normal organization skills, et cetera. Many have a higher than average expectation for their children; they look for ways to get the child into the best education systems, best learning places, among others.

When a parent finds out that their child has a hard time paying attention or learning, he/she may feel disappointed and maybe even feel guilty. It is important for the parent to understand that he/she is not the only one facing the issues; therefore, there is no need for guilt because he/she did not pass the struggles in behavior, directly or willing.

In some cases, the parent feels like he/she should do something to change the situation immediately, or that there is something that should have been done in order to prevent the condition. Understanding some of the drivers of this guilt and shame may help one to set aside their insecurities and take some good and positive steps for the better. Some of the reasons a parent feels guilty include:

- The feeling that the parent passed on the attention and learning issues to the child.
- The feeling that the parent overlooked the signs of the issue earlier.
- The feeling that a child should be normal and not have learning issues.
- The feeling that one is a bad parent, and other reasons.

For a parent, the most important part after learning that a child is dyslexic is finding ways to move past the emotions and expectations, and finding ways of helping the kid have a good life. The emotions and feelings are normal, the expectations that the child will get better or outgrow the challenges are normal. The guilt and shame affect a large number of parents for reasons that one can understand. However, these feelings might not be warranted or helpful. Some of these tips can help a parent set aside these feelings and become more productive for the child include:

Understand that you are not the cause of the issues that the child is facing.
As much as genes play a role in the attention and learning issues, it is not predictable. Some of the children in families that have signs of dyslexia may have difficulties, while some may not feel affected at all.

Some children will have the learning and attention challenges, yet they come from families with no history of dyslexia or ADHD.

Resist the desire to blame yourself or the other parent.
It is better if you work together and understand the condition of the child rather than pass the blame to one another.

Build a support system.
One of the things that help people facing common challenges is coming together and sharing ideas. Knowing that you are not facing an issue all alone helps a lot. Other parents and guardians who have children with dyslexia may offer valuable information and a listening ear. Family members may also offer help when they are aware of what the child is dealing with.

Know about learning, attention, and the specifics of your child as much as you can.
Understanding the specifics of the child and the learning rights can go a long way in boosting the confidence of the parent and the child. Besides, the knowledge will help you to set expectations within the right limits; therefore avoid disappointment. It also helps one to know what to ask for from the schools. Such knowledge is essential, because it helps one to realize that the child can get the right help and be successful and happy.

Have the strategies to cope with different life.

Some days are better than others with a dyslexic child. As such, one needs to find ways to keep from losing a temper and respond to the frustrations of the child and yourself. Staying calm and being empathic can help a parent to feel more in control and less torn about the reactions of the child.

Most importantly, a parent should have a plan to manage the circumstances that might trigger guilt or other emotions. Think of the best ways to respond to people who say things that might fuel the feeling of guilt or annoyance. Discover ways of working with other parties, for instance spouses, for the sake of the child.

Chapter 7: Your Child Just Needs to Learn Differently

As a parent or guardian of a child who has been diagnosed with dyslexia, it is important to understand that the kid is as active as the other kids of his/her age. The only difference is that they need different learning sessions. They may feel frustrated for being different from their peers. They might also feel some self-doubt, and if they are not supported well, the self-esteem may reduce. All kids want to be like their peers, and the dyslexic ones wish that their homework was as good as their friend's. They have a challenge completing the read and write tasks as effectively and beautifully as the other children. Consequently, they need help both at home and in school.

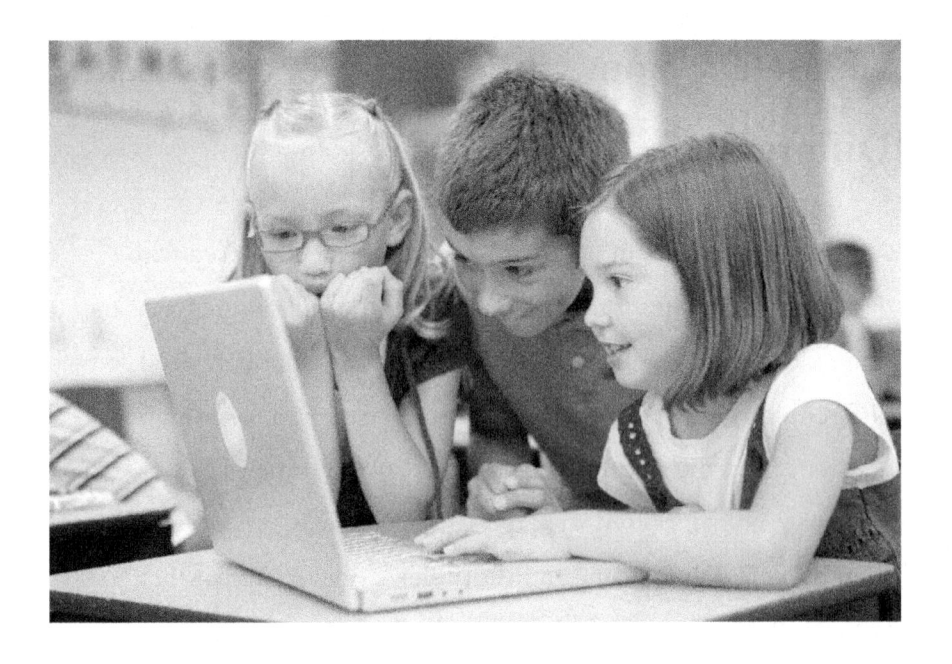

Of all the techniques that one will use to help the child learn, the main and most important is building the self-esteem of the child.

In school, it is important to ensure that the child gets the special learning guidance from the teachers. The parent may talk to the special needs teacher. Interestingly, most parents fail to talk to the teachers about the special needs of the child, because of the fear of putting labels on the kid or having the kid sidelined. Some parents cannot admit that the child needs extra help. It is important that one talks to the teachers in school even when overwhelmed. Early intervention of dyslexia is crucial for the child; therefore, if a parent suspects that the child has any difficulties learning, they should contact the school as soon as possible.

Researches have revealed that early intervention helps the child to build a positive image and maintain high self-esteem. It is better if the parent explains to the special education needs coordinator and teacher about the condition of the child. With the realization that the parent and teacher will need to do more in order to support the kid with most of the reading and writing tasks, it is important to keep an open communication channel.

Chapter 8: Test A Fish In Swimming But Not Climbing A Tree

No one put it better than Albert Einstein when he said that if one tests a fish by its ability to climb a tree; they will spend a lifetime thinking that it is stupid. In the real sense, a fish was not designed to climb trees; rather, it was given a special ability to swim. This illustration can be used when assessing the abilities of a dyslexic child. The solution is to identify the strengths and weaknesses of a kid and building on them. There are scientists who have spent most of their time identifying the advantages of having dyslexia, and they have found that although the dyslexic people do not have all the strengths, but each one has a unique pattern. Researchers Brock and Fernette Eide have found that dyslexic people excel more in four unique intelligence types, namely material reasoning, interconnected reasoning, narrative reasoning, and dynamic reasoning. In short form, the strengths are referred to as *MIND* strengths.

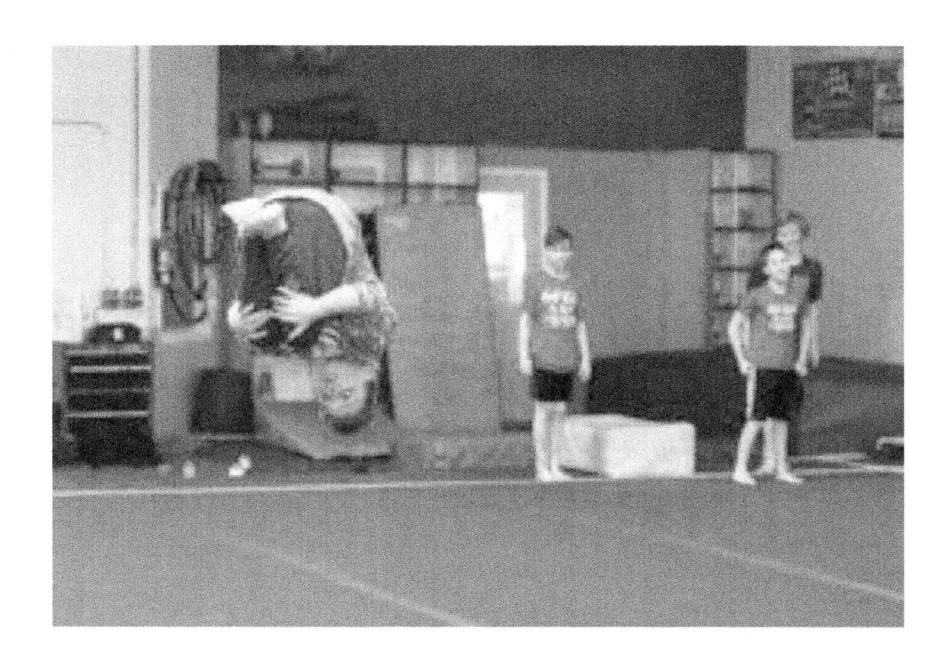

M - Material Reasoning

Material reasoning refers to the ability to apply visual-spatial relationships in three directional spaces. When put simply, Material Reasoning is the capacity to visualize and manipulate three-dimensional objects in the mind. As such, most dyslexic people are very good at activities such as engineering, architecture, and being artists.

I - Interconnected Reasoning

Interconnected reasoning refers to the ability to see the relationship between different concepts and things. Interconnected reasoning helps one to see the similarity of things. For dyslexic people, the reasoning enables them to see undiscovered and unique relationships between diverse concepts. This is one of the main keys of the creativity found in dyslexic people.

N - Narrative Reasoning

Narrative reasoning helps the dyslexic people to build a connected series of scenes in the mind to help recall the past, explain the things in the present, and to predict the future. In simpler terms, dyslexic people use stories to understand the world, and this explains why the majority of them are more gifted than normal people. This reasoning is also the key that allows the majority of the dyslexic people to remember complex details and put them into a story.

This explains why so many dyslexic people can remember many songs easily but forget things like phone numbers. Somehow the rhythm and rhyme of the song remind the dyslexic person of a story and he/she can visualize it while singing.

D - Dynamic Reasoning

Dynamic reasoning refers to the type of intelligence, whereby the person is able to predict the future with a certain degree of accuracy based on past data. This ability enables one to make real-life predictions based on complex data and observations. It takes many forms; for instance, an entrepreneur can collect some information about a business and predict the challenges and opportunities that might arise in the future. A geologist may be able to look at a formation of rock and imagine what they will look at in the next hundreds or thousands of years.

All in all, dyslexic people have a remarkable set of strengths and when identified early, the child can be taught how to build on it. The bottom line is to stop judging a fish by its ability to climb a tree. Stop focusing too much on the things that the child cannot do and look at what he/she is good at. Focus on what the child enjoys and help him/her get good at it. This will build confidence and self-esteem which will in turn flow over to other sectors of life.

Chapter 9: Self-Awareness And Acceptance For Kids With Dyslexia

When raising a dyslexic child, one will realize that the child thinks differently. The majority of dyslexic children are imaginative, creative, and tend to think outside the box. They are designers, builders, artists, junior entrepreneurs, and good storytellers. Many of the children diagnosed with dyslexia have a good memory for things that are presented in a logical way and have problem-solving abilities.

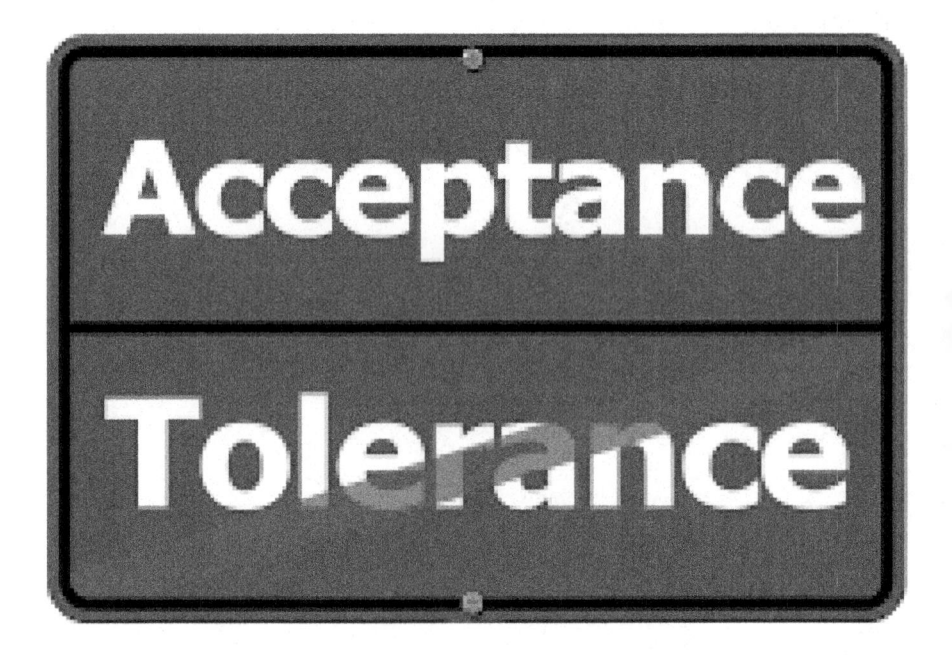

However, when raising a dyslexic child, you will notice that the child has a harder time learning to read, has trouble with punctuations and capitalization, is poor with spelling, and has poor handwriting. These children have challenges taking tests, putting their thoughts on paper, and demonstrating their knowledge in writing. Dyslexia makes one have problems with rote memorization and also remembering the sequence of handling daily tasks.

The brain of a dyslexic person is designed to do things differently compared to those without dyslexia. These people are able to see the big picture and think about it, get the gist of the situation, read situations and people, and identifying solutions that impact the masses. The catch is that we have to get the children who have dyslexia through school and also ensure that they feel good about who they are and their capabilities.

It is hard for a parent to watch their child suffer or struggle, especially if they did not go through the same challenge. A parent who has a learning disability has an easier time appreciate of why the child is having a hard time understanding things that are otherwise very easy. Those who have the same challenges also tend to wish that their child suffers less than they did. To complicate the issues, a parent may be re-living the school and childhood memories of reading struggle, and therefore are unable to help the child.

In most things related to parenting, it is important for the parent to be aware of their feelings and the triggers of the feelings, in order to be able to plan and figure out how to respond to a child. Having self-awareness and using the self-awareness to set apart the personal experiences from those of the child is important, because it helps the parent to support the child.

When raising a child with dyslexia, there are a number of things that a parent should focus on and consider. First, the parent should consider the strengths of the child. What do the kids like to do and what is of interest to them? What builds confidence and what makes the child lack self-esteem? The answers to such questions can help a parent to select the activities, mentorship programs, and life practices that will help the child to develop their skills and preferences, and to derive a stronger sense of the person they are.

The next essential step is to get support for the challenging areas. Dyslexic children would need more help in reading fluently, organizing words, and having better handwriting, learning how to stay organized, and understanding how their minds work best. These students will have better chances of learning if they can advocate for their own needs, for instance by explaining to the teacher what they need.

Another important thing is ensuring that the child gets the accommodation he/she needs to reduce the impact of the dyslexic style of processing in school settings. These children will need more time for writing, taking tests, and completing projects. They will also benefit more with tools such as keyboards, audiobooks, and dictation software. Again, the children will need a different technique of showing what they know, for instance by the use of oral presentations, oral tests and PowerPoints.

Healthy people are able to understand and own their weaknesses and strength. They are self-aware, and therefore are able to go through life with self-acceptance. It is important for parents and teachers to model self-awareness for children regardless of their condition, in order to help them accept and own who they are. Children tend to follow examples; therefore, it is important for parent or guardian to demonstrate self-acceptance and awareness in their own lives. Adults should show the children how to utilize their strengths and deal with the weaknesses by modeling perseverance and persistence. It is important to explain to the child that although it does not seem like it, dyslexia gives one an advantage over normal people. Their brain is designed differently for different things in an amazing way. Demonstrate to the child that it is possible to focus on the strengths and accommodate weaknesses by using these techniques in your life.

Chapter 10: Helping Your Child Breakthrough In Reading

As much as it sounds cliché, reading is a basic need in the world and one of the most important things that a parent can help a child achieve in order to get through life. The fact is—reading skills are needed in almost all aspects of life, from shopping to managing finances. Proficient reading is a basic tool for learning, and it is a large part of the subjects taught in schools. With the increased emphasis on literacy in education, one needs to help children to read, spell, and write down their thoughts. It is important to help a child with dyslexia to acquire adequate use of grammar.

Teaching a dyslexic child to read requires commitment, patience, and determination on the part of the parent and the kid. It is important to teach a child how to read from a tender age regardless of dyslexia.

Shared reading can go a long way in improving the reading skills of a child. Remember that dyslexic children are as intelligent and inquisitive as their peers and everybody else. As such, they enjoy things that other kids, do such as hearing stories. Reading to the child a story for at least 30 minutes a day can go a long way in uplifting all aspects of literacy skills. Re-read a favorite book, and although it might be boring for you, it will help the child to learn. The child does not even have to read by himself/herself in order to benefit; he/she needs to just be read to.

It is important to avoid putting pressure on the child while reading for them. Without pressure and with appreciation, the child will be able to pick more skills.

Start with simple books, such as picture books that have minimal to no writings. Make sure that the child relaxes and enjoys the story every day.

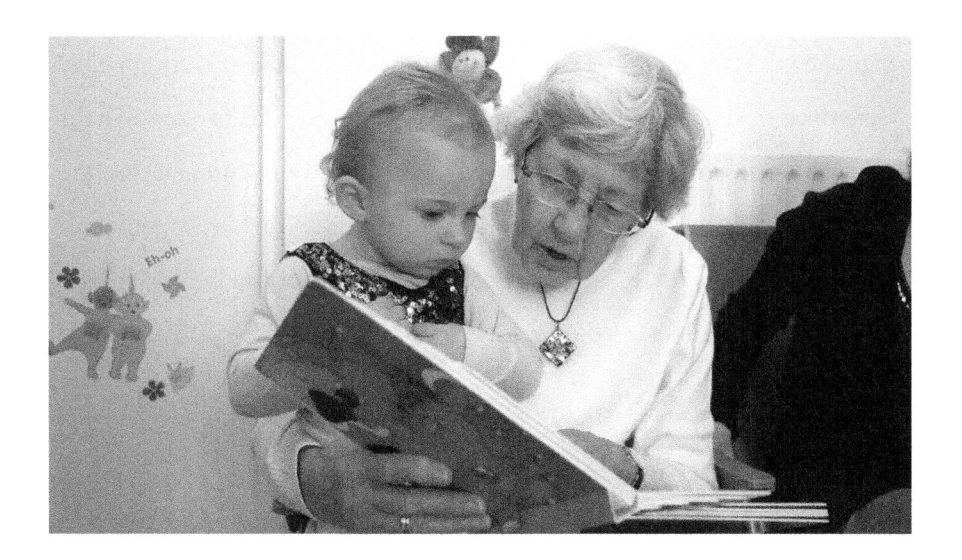

Simplified Steps

It is best if all parents start reading to their child at a tender age. Sometimes a parent might ignore a simple step like reading to a child with the assumption that the child will catch up when he/she gets to school. In fact, one current trend is that children spend more time watching television and playing video games than reading or participating in activities that might build their literacy skills. Starting early will help a parent to realize if the child has challenges and if there are ways through which he/she can help.

Encourage the child to read; begin with the simple words and sentences. After spending time reading stories to kids at a young age, take time to reverse roles. Encourage the child to read for you. The key to this achievement is praise. For every word or sentence that the child gets right, praise and congratulate the child. Early engagement with the child will help a parent to realize in time if the kid is dyslexic or having difficulties reading and writing.

Gradually Introduce Harder Books

A gradual choice of harder books will help the child to improve his/her literacy skills.

Try and share reading time with the child regardless of his/her age. This involvement will help the parent to observe the changes in the child. Further, the child will develop a deeper desire to read when he/she has the support needed.

Choosing the Books to Read

It is important to select books that create interest in the child. Beautiful illustrations and clear storylines are some of the things one should look for when selecting a book for the child. You can ask a teacher or dyslexia specialist for guidance on books that may help the child. Do not ask a child to read a book that is beyond their current level of skills. They will most likely feel demotivated. Motivation works best when the demands are not too high and the child can actually enjoy reading the book. A book that is beyond the skills of the child makes him/her labor, thus forgetting the meaning of what he/she is reading, and consequently, lose interest. The most important thing is to build the confidence and self-esteem of the child.

Handwriting

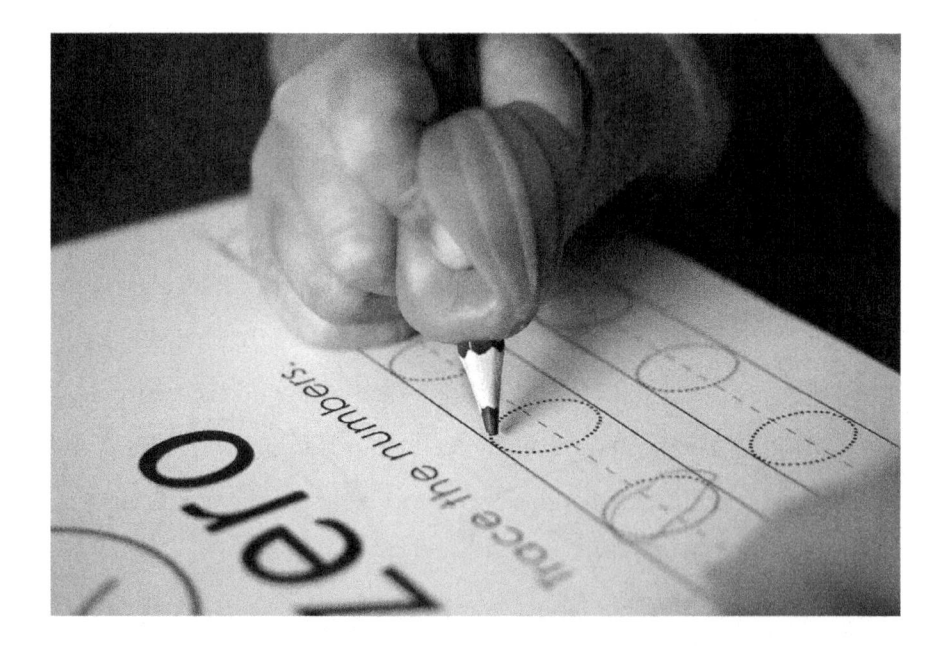

Another important part of literacy skills is handwriting. First off, handwriting is very important for self-esteem. Other kids can be unkind when talking about and dealing with kids who have messy handwriting. They may not understand the challenge behind bad handwriting, and as such, will make dyslexic children feel embarrassed.

Some of the ways that one can use to help the child have better and more organized work include:

- Using ruled and squared books and helping the child write within the lines.
- Giving the child a good pencil and eraser so that he/she can erase when the work gets messy.
- Reminding the child that writing needs both hands and concentration such that he/she holds the page down with one hand and writes with the other.
- Decorate the page, for instance using colors and stickers.
- Reward the child when the work is neat.

One may also use special tools such as pencil grip for the child. However, not all children who respond well to these tools; therefore, one should identify what works best for the kid. At a later age, a child may find it easier to type rather than write. It is not advisable to keep a child in front of a monitor for long hours. Building good handwriting takes time and effort. A technique that has been advocated to help a dyslexic child to read is the use of audio.

Chapter 11: Helping Your Child Breakthrough In Math

Math is a subject by itself, a language on its own and as such, it can present a lot of problems for the dyslexic child. It requires logical, conceptual, and spatial reasoning which are found on the right side of the brain, and most dyslexic children excel in this sector because they rely more on the right brain. It also requires exactness, neatness, and efficiency in computation skills, which are found in the left side of the brain. Some dyslexic children can be very good at math, but researches show that about 90% of the children with dyslexia have challenges with some areas of math. These children need to be explained the general terminology of math.

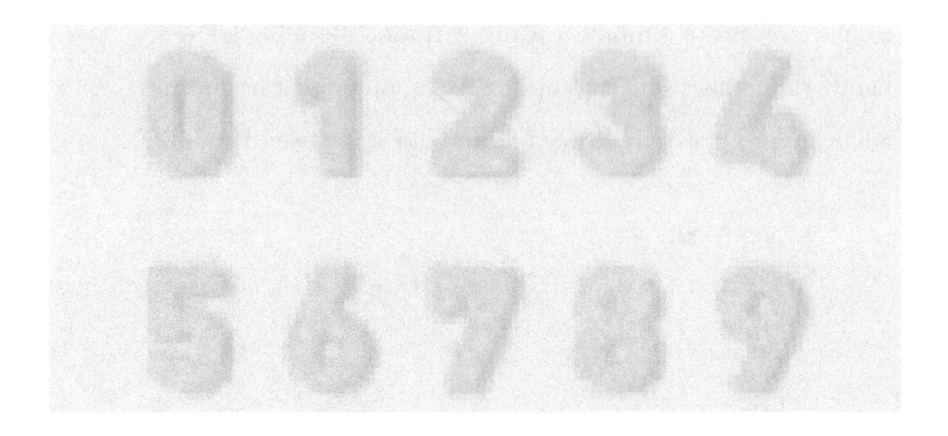

For instance, a child should know that the term plus, add, the sum of, total, and increase refer to single mathematical processes. Dyslexic children may also have a challenge with perceptual/visual skills, sequencing, directional confusion, memory, and word skills. They may also have difficulties with math problems that require a variety of steps, and those that place a heavy big load on the short term memory, for instance algebra or long division.

Techniques to Help a Dyslexic Child with Math

Using the Senses

The first thing that a parent and teacher should consider when teaching math to a dyslexic child is involving senses. Most of these children are visual; therefore, bringing in more visible content will help them utilize the strength. Kinesthetic learning will also help the child as he/she gets to do more than listen. The engagement of senses will help the child to concentrate and focus. Colorful objects such as toys, sticks, gemstones, et cetera, can help the child to connect the senses and grasp math.

Playing with numbers and objects will help to develop the learning abilities. The objective is to help the child combine different objects together to form a whole. Another way of incorporating physical activity into math is to use aids, such as skip counting, subtracting or adding.

Using Auditory Skills

Remember that dyslexic children have a good auditory ability; therefore, songs and rhythms can be a very useful tool for learning math. Naturally, children are drawn to rhyme and rhythm. A large number of good playground songs that people used to sing some years back are getting lost, and consequently, learning is becoming harder. These songs and counting games were very instrumental in the development of learning skills. Using rhyme and rhythms will help the child to develop his/her math capacity.

With dyslexic children, one cannot ignore the importance of the skills of estimation. A child should be taught and encouraged to use estimation. The child should also be taught to countercheck his/her answer against the question to see if the answer is sensible, possible, or ludicrous.

It is also advisable that the child uses verbal skills when doing math. This process involves verbalizing or talking through each step of problem-solving. A dyslexic child may also be encouraged to use a calculator as a way of proofing their answers.

In all cases, it is hard for one to learn while under stress. It is therefore important to build the self-esteem and confidence of the child, and ensure that he/she is not stressed.

Chapter 12: Seeking Therapy

Dyslexia is a result of issues with language, and the challenge normally begins with phonological awareness. This awareness is very essential for reading and as such, the children with poor phonological awareness having challenges recognizing and dealing with the sounds in words.

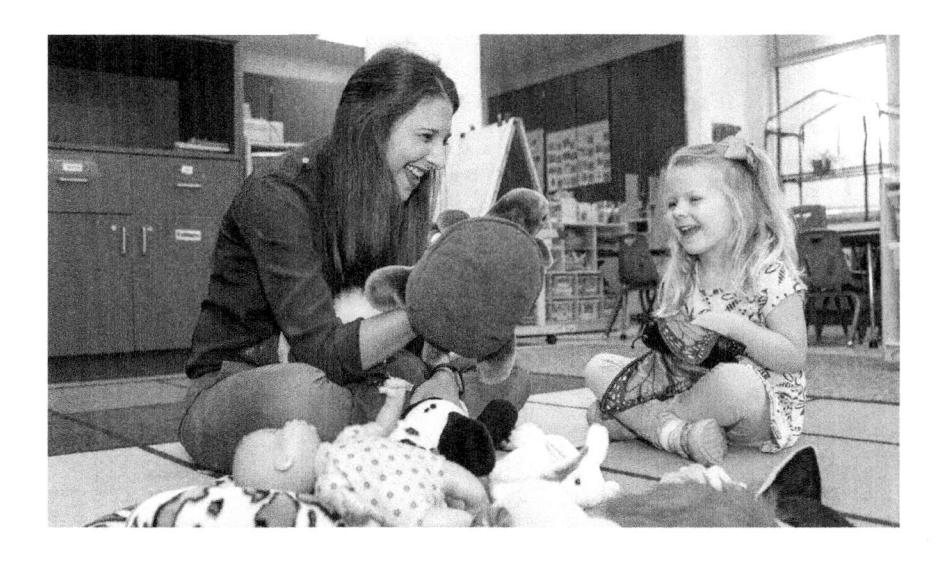

There are different types of therapy offered by specialists to help kids with dyslexia acquire literacy skills. The kids need to understand phonology and word sounds. These therapies help the dyslexic child to connect letters with sounds, blend sounds into words, and break words into sounds—phonics. When the skills are combined, they help the child to sound out the words they did not know. The process is referred to as decoding, and it is fundamental to reading. The professionals who offer this type of therapy include teachers, psychologists, reading specialist, speech-language pathologists, and learning specialists who focus on issues related to learning. These therapists work in schools and in a private setting. They build the phonological awareness of the child using various strategies, for instance by the use of rhymes and rhythms. They may help a child to remember the syllables by making them clap them out.

Specialists will generally look for ways to spot the best dyslexia treatment program with the stage that the child is in. After doing tests to assess how well the child reads or writes, the specialist will suggest the best-suited technique of dealing with the issue. Some of the intervention programs that a specialist may recommend include reading intervention programs, multisensory approach, and individual education plans.

Reading intervention programs are recommended to help build the skills of the student in terms of word recognition, spelling, and fluency. There are a number of programs available for the different students, and one of the most commonly used interventions is the Orton Gillingham program. This technique is research supported and has been used since the 1930s. It offers a multi-sensory structured education on language, whereby the children use touch, sight, and sound to connect the words and their sounds. The Wilson Language

Training and Preventing Academic Failure programs are based on the principles of Orton Gillingham.

The multisensory approach works because the primary objective involves helping the child to acquire stronger reading skills by using different senses. As such, most of the techniques used to adopt the use of a multisensory approach: touch, hearing, and visualizing. For instance, a teacher may use an exercise where the students tap out the syllables in the word in order to get the number. The teacher may also tell the student to trace out the shapes of the letters he/she hears. These exercises help the children with dyslexia to change the way they process information, therefore gradually improving their spoken and written language skills.

An individual education plan is a specialized instruction program that benefits the dyslexic children greatly. According to the federal law referred to as the Individuals with Disabilities Education Act, schools should take steps to help the children who have been officially diagnosed with dyslexia. The Individual Education Plan is a result of this law, and it provides accommodation to dyslexic children. The plan is normally developed by a team comprised of parents, the main teacher, school psychologist or any other dyslexia expert, a special education teacher, and a special education administrator. The specialists who diagnose and treat a child will most probably get into contact with the team to lay out an ideal IEP plan to help him/her succeed.

Technology for Older Children with Dyslexia
Many older children who have been diagnosed with dyslexia will feel more comfortable using computers and not exercise books. This comfort may be linked to the fact that a computer uses more of a visual environment that is better suited for the methods of learning used for dyslexic children.

Word processing programs are also very useful, because they have autocorrect and spellchecker facilities that highlight the typing mistakes for the child. Besides, the majority of the word processing software and browsers have text to speech functions that read the words as they are on the screen.

Speech recognition software can also be used to type out what the person is saying. Most of the dyslexic children have better verbal skills than writing skills; therefore, they may find the speech recognition software quite useful. There are also many other educational interactive software applications that will support the child by providing more engaging ways of learning.

Chapter 13: Joining A Support Group (Actually Helps)

Joining a support group has a variety of benefits, because it brings together people who are facing almost similar challenges. Feeling guilty, lonely, and scared things that most parents go through once they realize that their child is different. These feelings can form a vicious cycle for the parents; thus they need to identify the right support mechanisms. Support groups bring people together who offer each other moral support and emotional comfort. These people offer practical tips and advice to help one cope with the situation. The benefits of support groups include:

- Gaining a sense of control and empowerment.
- Feeling less isolated, lonely and judged.
- Adding to the sense of adjustment and improving the coping skills.
- Reducing depression, stress, fatigue, and anxiety.
- Letting one talk openly about their feelings without fear of judgment.
- Getting practical information or advice about the treatment options.
- Developing a clear picture of what to expect.

- Comparing notes about the condition.

Finding the Right Group

Finding a support group can be as challenging as finding a doctor or therapists. There are many options, but one has to identify the one that fits the specific needs. It may take a few trials for one to find an appropriate support group, but the best part is that there is a variety to select from.

There are three types of groups that are common, and they include local support groups, a personally started support group, and an online support group.

To begin a search, one can:
1. Search online for local international and social media based support groups.
2. Get recommendations from therapists, teachers, and other parties who might have the right information about such groups, among others.

Keep in mind that being a part of a support group involves connecting with other people and sharing essential information. You do not have to fit right in, and you have the right to take things slowly and focus on getting comfortable. Confidence in the support group is very important.

Understanding that one is not facing such a struggle alone helps both the parent and the child. It takes a lot of courage and trust to open up while there is a feeling of vulnerability.

Making a Financial Plan

A dyslexic child has special needs that need to be attended to. Schools are required to support children with learning disabilities, but the sad part is that not all of them have the resources required to do so comprehensively. Consequently, the parent will have to bear the cost of specialized education, outside tests, reading centers, and in some cases, private schools.

Some families spend more that tens of thousands of dollars to help the dyslexic children learn how to read before they can graduate from high school. Sometimes, one is faced with the challenge of saving up for college or helping the child to grasp the basics by hiring professional tutors. It is important to remember that if the child hates school and reading now, saving up for college will be of no benefit unless there are changes in the attitude. As such, one should give serious and deep consideration to what is best for the child.

Chapter 14: Summary: Ways A Parent Can Help A Dyslexic Child At Home

As a parent, you will be spending a lot of time with your child, and as much as you will feel confused, emotional, and guilty for the condition of the child, you will have to be strong for your child.

First, you need to be on the lookout for any signs of emotional stress in the child. The consequences of dyslexia can include frustration, low esteem, withdrawal, and anger. It is important that you find ways to make a child believe they are normal like their peers before you can help them build their literacy skills.

Second, children with dyslexia need continuous praise and support in order to build on self-esteem. It is important for everyone to have someone who believes and appreciates them. Let your child know that you appreciate and admire their efforts even if the results are not as good. It will have a positive effect on the mentality of the child toward reading.

Third, never compare the work of a dyslexic child with that of their siblings openly in a negative manner. A dyslexic child will already bad about himself/herself; therefore, comparing them with normal people will only ruin their confidence.

Fourth, do not lose your temper if a child losses a kit or forgets his/her homework. One of the consequences of dyslexia is that a child will forget where he kept things or the instructions he/she was given. They can hardly control the forgetfulness and will feel depressed and frustrated. As a parent, do not add on to the pressure by scolding the child. Instead, figure out ways to help him/her to be more organized.

Fifth, work together with the school teacher/educator. This will ensure that you know more about dyslexia, be able to keep track of new developments, and come up with comprehensive plans for helping the child.

Lastly, get the child assessed as soon as you suspect learning difficulties. It will help to rule out any other conditions and identify an early intervention plan.

Helping the Dyslexic Child with Organization

A child suffering from dyslexia will have a hard time organizing daily tasks and assignments. It is therefore important to identify strategies that will help the child to stay organized. Some of the strategies include checklists, routines, the use of color-coded timetables, planning things in advance, memorizing them, and establishing a place to put away things once you are done using them.

Helping a Dyslexic Child with Spelling

In most schools, the teachers teach spelling using the traditional method of look, cover, write, and check. However, this method does not apply for children with dyslexia.

The first step to helping the child spell is to pronounce the word as is spelled. For instance, if you are pronouncing the word 'want', say 'w-ant.' For a word that has silent letters such as 'Wednesday,' pronounce 'Wed-nes-day.'

The second step involves linking a word to a picture. A dyslexic child will more readily remember a picture because it is a visual clue. For instance, a child will forget that 'i' in the word 'first' and instead use 'e' as in 'ferst.' To remind him/her, draw an 'i' that is winning a race and say 'I comes first.' The child will remember the 'I' that won, thus remember 'first' and not 'ferst.'

The third step involves using a mnemonic. Mnemonics help the child to remember the spelling of a word. An example of mnemonic is, to remember the word 'does' one may say 'Does Oliver Eat Salad?' The first letter in each word represents a letter in the word we are trying to recall. Use a picture with the mnemonic to ensure that the child recalls more effectively.

Helping a Dyslexic Child with Writing

One of the most essential skills that everybody need in this world is to express thoughts on paper in a clear, understandable, and simple way. A dyslexic child will have challenges putting down their thoughts. In order to help them acquire this skill, you may read to them a story and tell them to retell it in the least words possible. These children also need more time than others to complete writing tasks.

One step to help the child put his/her ideas into words is to have a plan using keywords. Help the child to write down the keywords of the task as a guide for the idea. When the child gets to writing, he/she will just expand on the main word and strike it off the guide list.

The next step may be to ask their teacher to write down the homework for the child. Do the homework with your child and help them to write the words. In some cases, you may ask the school to accept typed out work from the child in order to help with spelling, speed, and legibility.

Helping a Child with Reading

It is important for you as a parent to support the child in reading. Some of the strategies that can help the child to read better include creating a thumbnail drawing on the margins of the book, besides the points. A dyslexic child will focus more on the mechanics of reading and forget the point that he/she has read. As a parent, assist the child to make the drawing that will help to remember the point.

You may also encourage the child to build up words by covering sections using a card or fingers. This will help the child to recognize suffixes and prefixes. Use colored backgrounds to help the child focus. Discuss the lessons you have learned after every reading session.

Helping Your Child with Memory

Majority of the children with dyslexia tend to think in pictures. You may use this strength to help the child remember things. Make page drawings to remember the main points. Avoid giving the child too many instructions at any one time.

Finally, ALWAYS reinforce the learning with multisensory activities and actions that are SEE it, HEAR it, SAY it, and DO it.

Conclusion

The moment a parent realizes that a child is dyslexic, a lot of things begin to make sense. Although the parent may feel guilty for the condition of the child, the knowledge enables him/her spot the ways to help the child. The parent also understands that he/she is not alone and the child is not the only one struggling. This book has taken you through the topic of overcoming dyslexia. It has used a simple language to help you understand the ways through which one can guide a child who has dyslexia.

Thank you for making it through to the end of this book, and we hope that the information found herein has helped you. Every effort was put to ensure that the chapters give you the necessary skills to help a dyslexic child. Just because you have completed the book does not mean that you have learned all there is to dyslexia. The only way to master dyslexia is by reading more and expanding the horizons.

The next step is to go and help a dyslexic child get better at reading and writing. You will realize that a good number of people do not know about dyslexia, so feel free to share the information you have acquired. If need be, join a support group, as it will ensure that you access more information. Pay attention to the changes that will take place in the child.

Jimmy D. Forest

Connect with us on our Facebook page www.facebook.com/bluesourceandfriends and stay tuned to our latest book promotions and free giveaways.

Printed in Great Britain
by Amazon